ESSENTIAL OILS USE AND SAFETY GUIDE FOR FAMILIES

Ninette Jackson, J.D., Certified Clinical Aromatherapist

Josiah's Oils is located at 8 Meadow Lane, Lancaster, PA and on-line at www.josiahsoils.com

*The information contained in this book is for educational purposes only. It is not meant to diagnose or treat any medical condition. The author is not a physician. <u>Always</u> seek medical advice from a licensed physician.

Genesis 1:11-12

Then God said, "Let the earth sprout vegetation, plants yielding seed, and fruit trees on the earth bearing fruit after their kind with seed in them"; and it was so. The earth brought forth vegetation, plants yielding seed after their kind, and trees bearing fruit with seed in them, after their kind; and God saw that it was good.

Essential Oils Use & Safety Guide

Introduction

By now most everyone has heard about essential oils. Recipes containing essential oils claiming to cure just about everything can be found on the internet. I have read many posts and blogs giving essential oils "advice," but dig a bit deeper into essential oils safety and you will soon learn that many social media claims regarding essential oils are simply unsafe. While some great resources do exist, it is important to navigate through the misinformation to find just the right balance. That is what I hope to offer in this book.

I am a Certified Clinical Aromatherapist and owner of Josiah's Oils, which has been serving the community with essential oils since 2011. I have vast experience working with clients in one-on-one consultations to find just the right oil blend suited for their particular needs. I have also lectured extensively concerning essential oils use and safety. I am a retired lawyer, wife, and the mother of five wonderful children, including Josiah after whom we named the company. Josiah is my precious gift of a son who happens to have Down syndrome. He benefits greatly from essential oils, thus we decided to name the company after him.

In all my years speaking about and working with essential oils, I have developed what I consider a very balanced and reasoned approach to using essential oils safely and effectively in your every day life. I do not exaggerate effectiveness, nor do I wish to cause such fear that oils are avoided. Instead, I like a safe and happy medium. Let's begin the adventure into safer essential oil usage!

Tiny, Healing Molecules

First, we will discuss what essential oils are and why they are so very popular. I always say that the power of essential oils lies in their weight - their molecular weight that is. The very small molecular weight of essential oils makes them readily absorbable and easily useful to the body.

We get essential oils usually by steam distilling fresh plants on farm. When we steam distill, we cause the cells of the plant to burst and release hundreds tiny of healing chemicals - natural ones that are specific to the plant distilled. These healing molecules (or constituents) are absorbed very readily into the body by inhaling or placing them on the skin, giving your body the direct healing benefits of the plant.

To get essential oils, we use parts of plants including seeds, roots, bark, stems, leaves, and flowers. The resulting essential oil contains some major constituents groups that can be generally classified as:

<u>Alcohols</u> - Antiseptic, antiviral, anti fungal, and up-lifting. [Examples: Palma Rosa & Tea Tree Oil]

<u>Aldehydes</u>- anti-fungal, anti-infectious, anti-inflammatory, immune-stimulating, antiseptic, calming to the nervous system; can be irritating to the skin (like lemongrass). [Examples: Lemongrass, Citronella, Cinnamon (true), Lemon Eucalyptus]

<u>Esters</u> - fragrant, anti-inflammatory, antimicrobial, relaxing and nourishing to the skin. [Examples: Lavender, Clary Sage, Bergamot, Sweet Marjoram, R. Chamomile, Frankincense.]

<u>Ethers</u>- similar in benefits to esters. [Examples: Anise, Basil, Cinnamon Leaf, and Fennel.]

<u>Ketones</u> - aid in removal of mucus, stimulate cell growth, relieve pain, may somewhat limit blood clotting, relaxes the mind. [Examples: Geranium, Spearmint, Rosemary, Helichrysum]

<u>Oxides</u> - anti-inflammatory, expectorants, anti-infectious, and analgesic. [Examples: Bay Laurel, Rosemary, Geranium, Eucalyptus *globulus*.]

<u>Phenols</u> - Strong anti-bacterial, Stimulating effect on nervous and immune systems, antioxidant, antimicrobial, anti-infectious, and may also help expel gas (may cause skin irritations). [Other examples: Oregano, Thyme, Clove]

Terpenes - May increase blood flow to the brain, anti-viral, anti-inflammatory, antiseptic, anti-fungal, protective of DNA, anti-allergen, expectorant, and supports detoxification. [Examples: Ginger, Citrus Fruits, Black Pepper]

Alkenes (a Terpene)- anti-inflammatory, well absorbed into the body, calming, relaxing, analgesic, protects cells, anti-fungal and antimicrobial [limonene is a common example, which is commonly found in citrus fruits like lemon as well as other oils].

All of these qualities sound impressive, but keep in mind that essential oil purity, distillation practices, proper farming and harvesting techniques, proper country of origin, storage history, and proper use significantly affect the therapeutic value of the constituents contained in essential oils. With regard to purity, use caution when purchasing essential oils as many oils on the market are tainted with: isolated synthetic compounds, synthetic fragrances, cheap essential oils, improper distilling practices, stretching chemicals, and other impurities. I have reviewed purity reports of oils at many "box stores", and they are nothing but chemical fragrances mis-labeled as "pure essential oils."

Even if some companies use *some* real essential oils, many use cheap alcohols, for example, to stretch a pure oil for greater profit. A plant may also be overly distilled to produce a cheap essential oil, thus negating its therapeutic benefits. As mentioned, synthetic fragrances are commonly added by companies to some common essential oils like lavender. Cheap Chinese cassia can be used by some less reputable companies in place of true cinnamon in blends which comes from Sri Lanka. The same holds true with cheap, less therapeutic lavender oils. Another popular trick companies use is adding cheaper similar-smelling oils to expensive oils to dilute them and increase profits. You do not want essential oils that have been altered by such dishonest practices. Be sure to purchase your oils from a trusted source with knowledge about safe usage. We strive to be that for our clients at Josiah's Oils.

Getting back to these powerful, tiny plant molecules: When we inhale essential oils the plant molecules are almost immediately:

1) absorbed by the lungs and nasal mucosa and then transported in the blood stream to the central nervous system where they act on neurotransmission; and

2) transmitted by the nose to the olfactory system which is connected with regions of the brain that control emotions and cognition (Limbic system). (See photo courtesy of MedScape)

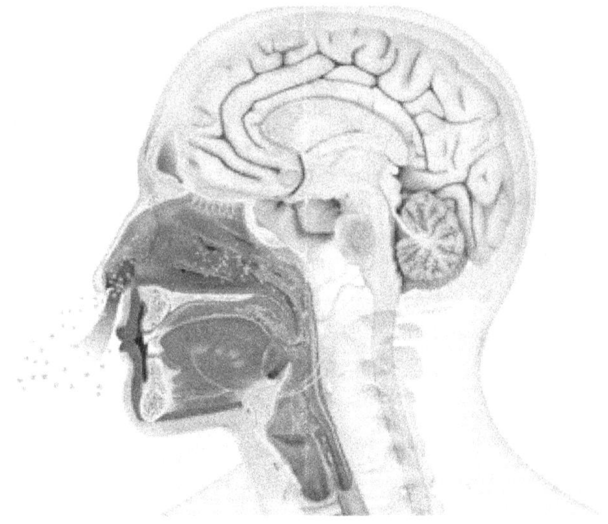

These olfactory and central nervous system connections are why essential oils can have an immediate affect on your emotions, your ability to concentrate, and on your congestion. [See <u>Quick Guide</u> in back of this book for the route essential oils take in the body after inhalation.] Many people, for example, enjoy inhaling rosemary essential oil in order to improve memory and focus. Thankfully, we don't need to rely on anecdotal stories of this working as science is catching up with nature and these types of responses are actually being documented.

Let's look at rosemary and the memory example. A 2012 study by *Therapeutic Advances Psychopharmacol* showed that performance and concentration on cognitive tasks improved <u>significantly</u> following exposure to diffused rosemary essential oil. [1] Inhalation is a simple way to enjoy the benefits of an

---

[1] Ther. Adv. Psychopharmacol. 2012; http://www.ncbi.nlm.nih.gov/pmc/articles/PMC3736918/

essential oil throughout your work or school day with a diffuser or personal inhaler.

In the brain's Limbic system is a complex system including the hypothalamus, hippocampus, amygdala, and Limbic cortex – which controls:

Hormone balance

Emotional Memories

Heart rate

Blood Pressure

Rapid Breathing

Memory

Learning

Emotions

Stress Levels

Hormone Balance

Release of neurotransmitters (Helps with focus!)

In my experience, diffusing is the safest and most effective way to use essential oils to infiltrate the Limbic System for emotional, memory, focus, or congestion related issues, and for killing airborne pathogens. (The other way essential oils can be beneficial to the body is topically applying essential oils to your skin, which will be discussed later in this book as well.)

Diffusing is simply the movement of molecules from a region of high concentration (in your essential oils bottle for example) to a region of low concentration (the surrounding air you breathe).

We can diffuse essential oils in a number of easy ways (see Quick Guide in back of this book):

- Simply taking deep inhalations out of the essential oil bottle. (In fact, essential oil molecules start to escape the moment you remove the cap!)

- Tenting, which is the process where one places about 6 drops of essential oil into a steaming water bowl and tents a towel over the head and deeply inhales. (always avoid the eyes and be careful of burns when tenting essential oils!)

- Palm inhalations, which is simply rubbing some diluted oils in the palm of your hand and cupping the mouth and nose and inhaling deeply.

- Applying oils to a personal inhaler (simply add drops to the container and place the cap on the inhaler, open, and inhale as needed.)

- Using oils in a therapeutic diffuser (water vapor or atomizing). Atomizing diffusers are the best for therapeutic uses as they diffuse only pure essential oil molecules. Whereas water vapor diffusers mix essential oils and water making the blend heavier which doesn't disperse *quite as well* into the air.

If using an atomizing diffuser, I generally recommend clients start by diffusing 2-3 times daily for about 20 minutes per session.*

TIP - Stronger Oils like cinnamon, clove, oregano . . . must be diluted well in a water diffuser and the time diffusing would be based on room size and dilution used; use caution when diffusing these oils in small quarters or higher concentrations. (See the

<u>Quick Guide</u> in the back of this book for details on factors to consider when diffusing oils.)

If you opt for a water-based diffuser, look for a diffuser that offers Mist Control (Low to High) and/or Intermittent Mist options. Such a mist diffuser can be used throughout the entire night for sleep issues or through the day for anxiety. A mist diffuser can also be beneficial for congestion adding moisture to the air along with the essential oils!

In your diffuser, excellent oils for sleep include lavender, bergamot, frankincense, valerian root, and cedarwood. Essential oils like eucalyptus, rosalina, rosemary, peppermint, and tea tree are excellent for diffusing in a water mist for congestion. We explore specific uses later in this book.

<u>TIP</u> - A couple of my favorite diffuser "recipes" are:

<u>Warm Pumpkin Latte 150 ml water add</u>:(You can easily turn this blend into a Gingerbread Latte with a few drops of ginger too!)

4 drops Coffee
4 drops Vanilla
3 drops Cinnamon
3 drops Clove

2 drops Nutmeg

<u>A Walk in the Autumn Leaves 150 ml water</u>:

6 drops Fir
4 drops Juniper Berry
4 drops Pine
4 drops Cinnamon

<u>Sunshine 100 ml water</u>:

6 drops Lime (or Key Lime)
4 drops Geranium

<u>Sinus Buster 150 ml water</u>:

4 drops Peppermint
4 drops Eucalyptus
2 drops Cypress
4 drops Lemon

<u>Pick-Me-Up 100 ml water</u>:

4 drops Palmarose
4 drops Lavender
4 drops Tangerine

In addition, essential oil diffusers have the added benefit of being ionizing to the air in your home or office - especially atomizing models. Indoor air contains large quantities of positive ions, which are simply atoms that have a <u>positive</u> electrical charge because they contain more protons than electrons. This is caused largely by things like computers, cell phones, and other electronics in the home. These positively charged ions can cause fatigue, headaches, and other health issues. Negative ions added to the air by essential oil diffusers on the other hand help to increase energy and physical activity.

Diffusing isn't the only way to enjoy essential oils. We will now examine topical applications, which also produce amazing results.

Carrier Oils

Before an essential oil may touch your skin, you must dilute it in a carrier oil. Unlike an essential oil, a carrier oil is a fatty - or fixed - oil. I love the term "carrier" because it illustrates what the fatty oil does to the essential oil: it carries or envelopes it - like a little package of health! Why must we diluted in a fatty oil? It is because essential oils are lipid soluble, not water soluble. This means is you "mix" water and oils, the oils will simply "sit" on top of the solution.

Unfortunately, it is becoming increasingly popular to use essential oils without dilution (or neat); in most cases, with the exception of very few oils such as true lavender (*l. angustifoila*) for specific *limited* needs, this practice is not safe!   For example, oregano oil can cause severe burns on the skin if applied neat. Even gentle oils like lavender, if misused by continually applying neat to the skin begin to cause contact irritation over time and can cause a development of an allergy to that oil.

Getting back to carrier oils, these oils contain fatty acids, fat soluble vitamins, minerals, and other essential nutrients. Fatty acids in carrier oils not only provide protection for the skin, but they also help strengthen the skin and reduce appearance of fine lines/wrinkles. Some carriers like jojoba, have anti-inflammatory properties. So carrier oils can have their own added bonuses to both your skin and your overall health.

TIP- If you spill undiluted essential oils on your skin "wash" them off with a carrier oil or other fatty liquid, which can immediately provide fatty dilution to the area minimizing the damage. Do this as soon as possible.

Carrier Oils are also known to extend the therapeutic action of the essential oil as they lengthen the time the aroma is present for the olfactory system response - thus they are beneficial for emotional uses as well as the tissue.

It is important to note that some carrier oils oxidize quickly. Indeed, many can go rancid and expire in about 3-6 months. Thus, it is important not to create blends containing carriers and essential oils in large batches.

TIP- Carrier oils should be stored in a cold, dark place. Preferably the refrigerator. (They may get cloudy in cold storage, but you may simply return the carrier to room temperature to stabilize before use.)

A few good options for carrier oils include:

<u>Grapeseed</u> - benefits:

- Gentle

- Moisturizing

- Odorless

- Readily absorbed

- Contains potent antioxidants that protects against cellular and tissue damage

- Contains vitamin E

- Helps heal wounds and scars

- Will not clog pours

- Anti-inflammatory

<u>Jojoba</u> (Golden) - Benefits:

- Liquid ester similar to the one in human skin and not actually an "oil", but a liquid wax

- Penetrates rapidly

- Doesn't go rancid quickly

- Balances PH

- Will not clog pores

- Great for acne as it reduces build up of sebum

- Anti-bacterial

- Promotes hair growth

- Mimics collagen

- Anti-inflammatory

Fractionated Coconut Oil (liquid) - benefits:

- Nourishing to the skin

- Contains antioxidants

- Provides protective barrier

- Long shelf-life

Sweet Almond - benefits:

- Easily Absorbed

- Contains Vitamins A, B1, B2, B6, D, & E

- Good for dry, sensitive, or inflamed skin

- Good for eczema, psoriasis, and dermatitis

As you can see, there are many other carriers oils from which to choose. My personal favorite during my years working with clients is Jojoba due to its ability to penetrate deeply and its long shelf life. Once you select your carrier oil, you then need to know how to add the essential oil into the carrier before you apply to the skin. There are two ways to do this:

1. You may make up a blend in advance and keep it in an essential oil bottle (like cobalt blue or amber glass); or

2. You may mix the blend in your hand with each use.

Either way, we call mixing the essential oils and carrier oils a dilution. Dilution ratios do not change whether you mix in a bottle or your hand. Some like to mix-as-they-go so they are not committed to an entire container of a blend. It is also helpful to mix in your hand as the oils get well blended and application can be in the form of massage. To do this simply take your less

dominate hand and place about a teaspoon of carrier oil. Then

grab your essential oil and add your drops. Your dominate hand is

then free to apply the mixture to the place most needed.

Whichever way you decide to do it, the next step is to know your

oil's dilution needs.

Dilute, Dilute, Dilute

Just like foods, people can react to different plants in

different ways. If you eat too much of a strong spicy food - you

might get ill - even burns in your mouth and esophagus. The same

holds true with oils; but to an even greater degree due to their

concentrated nature. Some essential oils are <u>far</u> more likely to

cause a reaction than others and we should know which those are.

Examples of commonly irritating essential oils are oils high

in phenols. It is common for people to be sensitive to larger

amounts of phenols even in foods. Phenols are extremely anti-

microbial, but can burn the skin and possibly mucus membranes if misused (overused or not diluted properly). Oils that may cause

this reaction include:

Cinnamon (all types), Clove, Oregano, Thyme (to name the

most commonly used) [2]

Whichever oil you select, proper dilution is <u>key</u> to safely in

using essential oils. Many oils that are highly sensitizing require

maximum dilution of .5% or 1%. That means for each teaspoon of

carrier you would calculate the amount of essential oil. At Josiah's

Oils, we place the proper dilution ratio on each bottle so there is

an easy reference point when mixing.

Sensitivity can develop over long term use. Those who have a
history of allergy symptoms like asthma, eczema, or hay fever
need to use extra caution. Also, sometimes a mixture of essential
oils can trigger a reaction. Proper dilution aids in reducing the
risk of sensitization!

The easiest equation is:

1 teaspoon carrier plus 1 drop of oils = 1%

To get .5% you need to add one drop of essential oils to 2 teaspoons of carrier oil.

There are 30 ml in 1 ounce, so our 2 teaspoon example is 10 ml or 1/3 of an ounce. Other exact percentages can be computed from the standard equation above. For example, .5% can also be estimated by simply taking 4 teaspoons of carrier oil (or 20 ml) and adding 2 drops of essential oil. (These lower dilutions are useful for younger children.) Here are some helpful guidelines:

Per 5 ml (1 tsp.)	1 Drop Essential Oil	= 1% Dilution
Per 10 ml (2 tsp)	1 Drop Essential Oil	=.5% Dilution
Per 15 ml (3 tsp)	1 Drop Essential Oil	=.25% Dilution
Per 5 ml (1 tsp.)	2 Drops Essential Oil	= 2% Dilution
Per 10 ml (2 tsp)	2 Drops Essential Oil	= 1% Dilution

Per 15 ml (3 tsp)   2 Drops Essential Oil   =.50% Dilution

Per 5 ml (1 tsp.)   3 Drops Essential Oil   = 3% Dilution

Per 10 ml (2 tsp)   3 Drops Essential Oil   = 1.5% Dilution

Per 15 ml (3 tsp)   3 Drops Essential Oil   =.75% Dilution

Per 5 ml (1 tsp.)   4 Drops Essential Oil   = 4% Dilution

Per 10 ml (2 tsp)   4 Drops Essential Oil   = 2% Dilution

Per 15 ml (3 tsp)   4 Drops Essential Oil   = 1% Dilution

TIP- Most common roller bottles used to make essential oils blends hold 10 ml, or two teaspoons.

TIP - Essential oils bottles generally come in 5 ml (1 teaspoon), 10 ml (2 teaspoon), or 15 ml (3 teaspoon) size options.

When using essential oils topically, covering the area after application will help with absorption due to the volatility of the oil, which is just a fancy way of saying the oil likes to escape into the air. Also, more frequent application may assist with absorption when coving the area is impractical. For stomach pain and cramping, for example, I recommend applying a diluted oil like Clary Sage and then covering with a warm (not hot), moist pad for deep penetration.

Next, it is always important to perform a patch test for allergies or sensitivities before using a larger amount of oils on the body if you are sensitive. This way you can gauge which essential oils, if any may cause a reaction for you. To do this:

*Take one drop of essential oil and one drop of carrier oil then apply to wrist or forearm covering with a bandage; check in a few hours, but ideally you would leave on for a full 24 hours; when you remove the bandage look for itchiness, redness, burning, irritation. (*do not attempt patch testing without medical supervision if you are a highly allergic individual.)*

Do not attempt this type of patch testing with the highly irritating oils we have discussed as redness would occur on any skin-type. For those oils add a drop of essential oil to a teaspoon of carrier oil, mixing well before testing. You may select an area of the skin to test that is not visible such as behind the knee and add a drop to the area after mixing.

To evaluate the results of patch testing, know that red, irritated skin indicates that a specific essential oil should be avoided. While many will claim a skin reaction to essential oils is part of the detoxification process, actually the use of any such oil should be discontinued following a reaction. Depending on the severity or response, reapplication at a later time with a greater dilution might be appropriate.

For the most part, proper dilution of most essential oils for the skin is considered to be 5% (or 5 drops per teaspoon of carrier oil), but there are many exceptions. Sore muscle recipes, for example, are generally made at a 20% dilution ratio. That is 20 drops per teaspoon of carrier oil. Another exception, essential oils used on the face are usually limited to a 1% dilution ratio and one must always avoid the eyes. (See <u>Quick Guide</u> to safe Dilution in back of this book)

There are some other key safety issues to be mindful of when using essential oils, which we will explore now.

Blood Pressure

Some essential oils (notably rosemary, eucalyptus, and perhaps peppermint) *might* raise blood pressure. Use essential oils with caution on those with a history of high blood pressure. I note there is little evidence to support this and many people who have high blood pressure (myself included) can use these oils without difficulty; just take caution for the rare chance that individuals may have increased blood pressure following use of certain essential oils. Due to the even slightest potential, it would be prudent to check your blood pressure results after using these essential oils a few times and (as always) consulting with your physician if you suffer from HBP that isn't well controlled.

Seizures

Seizures

All who have a history of epilepsy or are taking anti-seizure medications must use extreme caution with oils. The constituents in essential oils to avoid completely include: camphor, methyl salicylate, pinocamphone, cineole, sabinylaceate, fenchone, pulegone, and thujone. Oils containing some of these constituents include: eucalyptus, rosemary, fennel, wintergreen, sweet birch, and hyssop. There are also other less common oils to avoid. *Always consult with a certified clinical aromatherapist and most importantly with your physician before using oils if you suffer from a seizure condition.

Out with the Old (Expired Oils and Storage)

Use extreme caution with old essential oils. Freshness is far too often overlooked with regard to safety and therapeutic uses of essential oils. Many essential oils over a year old can irritate the skin due to oxidization, which is described below. Thus, old oils are only good for cleaning purposes, but should not be used therapeutically. As mentioned, we now see essential oils for sale in almost every box store. I can't imagine these oils are remotely fresh as they must sit in warehouses, trucks, stores. . . for an extended time period with unregulated (often extremely hot) temperatures.

Thus, the first concern is buying oils you know are truly fresh. This brings us to the issues involved with how to *keep* your essential oils fresh and pure. Light, heat, and/or air can cause certain chemicals in essential oils to oxidize or change and become irritating to the skin. (This process is called oxidization.)

Because the active constituents oxidize into harmful chemicals, the essential oil loses it therapeutic effect over time. Never make a cleaning solution combining essential oils with hydrogen peroxide for this reason.

Some important guidelines to follow to ensure the highest therapeutic oils:

1. Buy Fresh. Buy only fresh oils that are kept in <u>cold storage</u> and sold fresh with little time between distillation and bottling/sale.

2. Keep Cold. Cold storage can extend the life of an essential oil by 2-5 years and keeps the essential oils far fresher <u>before</u> you even bring them home. Why buy oils that have been left in heat and damaged even before you bring them home? *always keep oils under 65 degrees even if you do not refrigerate.

2. Tighten Up. Tightly replace caps after each and every use and store them in proper glass containers (see #3).

3. The correct color. Amber glass (not blue) is best as it lets in less UV rays.

4. Wait to mix. Once mixed with fatty carrier oils essential oils may turn rancid faster and much be used within 3 to 6 months (unless a longer lasting carrier oil is used like Jojoba).

5. Refrigerate. Store essential oils known to oxidize quickly in the refrigerator, unless you plan to use them within 6 months to 1 year. This includes all citrus oils, tea tree, and lavender. I like to use a container (like a food storage with a lid) so the food in my refrigerator does not smell like essential oils. I note that a few essential oils actually get better with age; examples include sandalwood, patchouli, and frankincense.

6. Protect. Never leave essential oils in sunlight, steam, or heat. Never store essential oils in the bathroom with a bath or shower. Never leave them in the car on warmer days or on window sills.

7. Toss. Discard old bottles that have not been properly stored if those oils have been opened over 12 months prior or distilled long ago; alternatively, you may use those oils for cleaning.

TIP-Toilet sprays are a great idea for older essential oils; simply add 20 drops of an oil like Tea Tree and/or Lemon to a 2 ounce spray bottle filled with distilled water and spray before you go. You can leave a bottle in the powder room with a cute label like Poo Poo Potion Spray.

8. Do not use bottles with rubber tops and droppers as the rubber leeches into the oils.

9. Place dates on the bottles (dates you purchased and opened). Small, round labels are perfect for this.

Sun Exposure

The next safety concern to address is sun exposure. Photosentization is a reaction to something applied to the skin that occurs in the presence of UV light. (Without UV light these chemicals are not damaging to DNA.) The resulting damage is called Photo-contact dermatitis. The fairer skinned the person, the higher likelihood of this type of dermatitis.

SKIN + THESE OILS + ULTRAVIOLET PHOTONS (NATURAL OR IN A SUN BED) = CAN PRODUCE A BURN REACTION

ESSENTIAL OILS KNOWN TO BE PHOTOTOXIC

BERGAMOT*

FIG ABSOLUTE

LEMON*

LIME*

BITTER ORANGE

RUE

ANGELICA ROOT

CUMIN

GRAPEFRUIT

*expressed oil only; steam distilled versions are not photo-toxic
*Josiah's Bergamot is not photo-toxic as it is bergaptene-free

Lime oil is a serious photosensitizer. If you are making a blend for someone who spends time in the sun please use caution and use these guidelines:

- There is little to no risk if essential oils are used in a wash off product like shampoo or wash;

- Combining photo-toxic oils increases risk (for example a lemon and lime blend);

• The risk for reaction increases the first hours after

application, then decreases slowly thereafter;

• When using an essential oil known to be photo-toxic, avoid

UV light for 12-18 hours following use on exposed skin!

Bathing

Next, bathing with essential oils can be a relaxing experience, but please consider some safety guidelines. First, be careful to select gentle oils and disperse in bath before you enter. A great choice is lavender before bed. Add a few drops of a fatty carrier oil to the essential oils and mix well before dispersion. This will add the benefit of softened skin. Also be careful of slips and falls as the carrier will make the bath slick!

Blood Thinning Oils

Even inhalation can cause the essential oil you are using to enter your blood stream, so it is important to use caution with regard to any essential oil if you are on blood thinning medication, or if you are planning to have surgery. The oils that are known to inhibit blood clotting are:

Birch (Sweet), Garlic, Oregano, Tarragon,

and

Wintergreen

However, many other oils _may_ inhibit blood clotting. These include oils like cinnamon and clove. It is best to check with a professional regarding the specific oil you wish to use when you are taking blood thinning medication and to avoid them if you are planning surgery.

Should I Eat and Drink my Oils?

We all know someone who loves to drink their oils in water, right? It is very important to note that *all* major aromatherapy organizations do not recommend internal use unless you are working with a trained professional. Damage can result to the esophagus, stomach, and liver. Internally used essential oils can also contradict medications.

As discussed, essential oils need to be treated with great care. Indeed, ingestion of only a teaspoon (5 ml) of eucalyptus oil can be fatal to a child - same with wintergreen oil at even lesser amounts. In addition, lemon essential oil contains high amounts of Limonene - a solvent that can damage your esophagus.

TIP - If you have doubts as to the solvency power of lemon essential oil try this little test. Place a drop or two of lemon essential oil on a tissue and wipe off a scribble made with a permanent marker (use caution not to ruin the surface you are testing).

Have you noticed that the people who drink their citrus oils like lemon in water know they need to use a glass or stainless steel bottle, not plastic due to power of the essential oil to "eat through" plastic. If the essential oils are too harsh for plastic, imagine the potential damage to your sensitive digestive track.

A 2015 study by the Atlantic Institute of Aromatherapy revealed that most essential oils injuries occurred when essential oils were used neat (undiluted) or when taken internally. Tellingly, no adverse reactions were reported when clients worked with a properly trained, certified aromatherapist.[3]

This is not to say you may *never* use some safe oils internally. Working with a trained medical professional knowledgeable in essential oils is important. You should review a detailed history of your medications looking for potential contradictions or reactions as well as knowing which oils are toxic and which are not. Not the kind of information you want to trust social media to answer![4]

Finally, water is never a "carrier" safe for any internal uses as it lacks fat. Instead, a carrier oil or honey is a better choice to protect the sensitive digestive track when taking essential oils

---

[3] To read the full report: http://aromatherapyunited.org/injury-reports-february-2015/

[4] Ingestion safety and oil purity are not the same. Ingestion caution is <u>purely</u> a safety issue.

internally. In addition, capsules are generally needed for internal uses of essential oils. As you can see, drinking drops of essential oils in water would never be safe.

Some oils have been given GRAS status by the FDA. This simply means they are "Generally Regarded as Safe." At Josiah's Oils we state "GRAS" under the description of these oils so they are easy to identify without heading the the FDA's website. (See our <u>Quick Guide to GRAS</u> essential oils in the Quick Guide Section of the book. I note that although Hyssop is included by the FDA, I have seen reports of toxicity from that oil and I would not recommend using it internally.) The FDA specifically notes that the list does *not* mean that the oils have been acknowledged as safe as supplements, only that they are considered safe for consumption in historic/commonly-used amounts to flavor foods.

We know that many of these GRAS oils can be used in safe ways to enhance flavors when cooking. An example would be adding one or two drops of lemon essential oil to a fatty cooking oil, like coconut. After this you can add your chicken or other protein and have lemon chicken. You can make orange chicken in a similar way. To disperse the flavor however be sure to add the essential oil to the fatty oil in your dish. These GRAs oils can also be used to make a salad dressing. Add a drop or two of grapefruit to 4 ounces of olive oil, then add vinegar makes a delicious salad dressing! Honey is another safe "fat" for diluting essential oils as food flavorings. Just remember with flavoring, more isn't always better. A drop of essential oil in a few ounces of fatty cooking oil or honey usual does the trick! (See the <u>Quick Guide</u> for a few more recipe ideas!)

Essential Oils & Children

How old should a child be before using essential oils on their skin? Many people feel it is safest to await topical application until a child is 24 months. Younger skin absorbs essential oils at far greater rates. Before the age of 2, diffusing certain essential oils in a safe and proper proximity to the child is considered safer than topical use. There are some oils to avoid; the information below concerning eucalyptus, rosemary, and peppermint from the

Tisserand Institute proves helpful:

- Eucalyptus & Rosemary – MAY diffuse at 6 months with 1% dilution ratio (no topical uses at this age).

- Peppermint – NO topical uses until 3; avoid diffusing until 3; until the age of 6 keep dilutions at 1% (See <u>Quick Guide</u> with this information at the back of this book)

<u>TIP</u>- For recipes using eucalyptus or rosemary you can safely switch to fir essential oil (absent allergies of course).

<u>TIP</u>- For recipes calling for peppermint, you can safely use Spearmint (absent allergies).

I should note I do not agree with websites that claim these oils are absolutely unsafe for children under 10. There is no evidence to support this theory and I believe the Tisserand Standard described about is abundantly cautious. Next, if you do decide to use essential oils topically under the age of two, try to avoid skin irritating oils (those considered typical skin irritants) or use much greater caution if using these particular oils on the skin:

Clove, Cassia, Lemongrass, Ylang Ylang, Thyme, Oregano

Prior to the age of 2, if you decide to diffuse oils, do so at a safe dilution in your water vapor diffuser and at safe distance away from the baby. You may also stick with the essential oils on the *Kid Safe List* below.

It is important to know that certain oils are toxic if ingested *and* may be toxic even if too much is applied to the skin. These oils *must never* be used on children. For example, *Methyl salicylate* (an ester found naturally in Wintergreen and Sweet Birch) is extremely toxic to the body in higher concentrations. In 2007, an athlete died at age 17 after <u>absorbing</u> too much of a muscle pain relief product containing *Methyl salicylate.* (This product was *not* an essential oil but a solution of the concentrated *Methyl salicylate*.)[5]

Kid-Safe List

Thankfully there are many oils to select that are generally considered safe to use on children! Here is a list of examples of some (not all) common *Kids Safe* essential oils for the *younger* children in your life (usually 3 and under):

Bergamot

Black Pepper

Blood Orange

Cedar wood

Clary Sage

Copaiba Balsam

---

[5] Hyssop is another oil that may be toxic if misused and thus should be avoided in children.

Coriander/Cilantro

Cypress

Frankincense

Chamomile

Geranium

Ginger

Grapefruit

Juniper Berry

Helichrysum

Ho Wood

Lavender

Lemon

Mandarin

Neroli

Palmarosa

Patchouli

Petitgrain

Pine (Scotch)

Rosalina

Sandalwood

Siberian or White Fir Needle

Spearmint

Spruce

Sweet Marjoram

Sweet Orange

Tangerine

Tea Tree

Vetiver

Josiah's Happiness Blend

Josiah's FOCUS Blend

Josiah's Sniffles Congestion Blend

Josiah's Kids' Blend INSECT AWAY

Josiah's Immune Boost

Josiah's Germ Stopper Blend

Josiah's Kids' Calm

Josiah's Bite Repair

Josiah's ZZZs Blend

Josiah's Worry Less Blend

Josiah's Sore Tummy Blend

For these safer oils, we still want to use safer dilution ratios for topical applications on much younger children. The younger the child, the higher the dilution - starting with .25% is usually best. (4 teaspoons of carrier oil to one drop of our safe essential oil is .25%). If tolerated and as the child gets older, you may increase up to 5% depending on the age of the child *and* the oil used.

A fun and safe night-time calming recipe (for most children) is a room spray. Mix 2 ounces of distilled water with 10 drops of Lavender, 5 drops of Bergamot, and 3 drops of Cedarwood. (Be sure to shake well before each use!) This blend should produce a pleasant night's sleep when sprayed in the air of the room before bed.

If you have small children in your home and an essential oil collection, always keep the number for poison control on hand. The American Association of Poison Control Centers has an *extensive database* of essential oils and can assist Emergency personnel when called. The Association supports the nation's 55 poison centers in their efforts to prevent and treat poison exposures. Poison centers offer free, confidential medical advice 24 hours a day, seven days a week through the Poison Help line at 1-800-222-1222.

It is also helpful to keep activated charcoal (capsule) on hand to swallow if needed. Activated charcoal contains many small chambers and cavities that bind-up unwanted material and protects the body from overdosing on harmful toxic substances. Do not however use charcoal instead of calling a medical professional.

A Word on Pets

I recommend that you never diffuse in a small room with a caged animal (lizard, hamsters, birds, fish, rabbits, mice…). These pets cannot express if they feel ill (headaches, stock ache ache and so on). Cats lack the liver enzymes to properly break down the essential oils in their body so never use Essential Oils on cats. Due to their highly sensitive metabolic systems, cats and essential oils do not mix! If you diffuse and own a cat, allow for a means of egress for the cats into an area where <u>no</u> oils are being used/diffused. Large dogs and farm animals usually love Essential Oils and process them well, but consider Kids Safe oils (see the list in the Use & Safety guide and on Josiah's Oils bottles where there will be a Kids Safe Logo) for them when diffusing and always talk to your vet.

Pregnancy & Essential Oils

Many moms avoid topical use of essential oils during the first trimester. After this, we have a list of examples of oils that are considered safe for use during pregnancy in proper dilution:

Bergamot

Blood Orange

Copaiba Balsam

Coriander/Cilantro

Cypress

Siberian or White Fir Needle

Frankincense

Grapefruit Citrus

Ho Wood

Helichrysum

Juniper berry

Lavender (specifically *Lavandula angustifolia*)

Lemon

Mandarin

Neroli Citrus

Pine (Scotch)

Sweet Orange

Tangerine

Thyme

Josiah's Happiness Blend

Josiah's Sniffles Blend

Josiah's FOCUS Blend

Josiah's immune Boost

Josiah's Kids' Calm

Josiah's ZZZ's

Josiah's Worry Less

Josiah's Germ Stopper

Other essential oils not on the list above also may be OK to use, *if* properly diluted. Consult a qualified aromatherapist regarding specific oils not mentioned as there are hundreds of different essential oils on the market today. Start with .25% to 1% dilution and evaluate what is tolerated. Avoid essential oil applications directly over the stomach during pregnancy as well and always consult with your obstetrician. Properly diffusing essential oils is generally considered safe in pregnancy.

Morning Sickness

Essential oils can be a great help during pregnancy. A 2014 randomized clinical trial showed a "significant" decrease in nausea and vomiting in the 100 pregnant women who inhaled lemon essential oil! These pregnant women had suffered from nausea and vomiting during their pregnancy before using the essential oil. Thus, lemon oil might be a safe and effective oil to have on hand if you suffer from morning sickness. [6]

TIP - You can create a Morning Sickness Inhaler by taking a personal inhaler and adding a few drops of both lemon and ginger essential oils. Inhaling preventatively is always a good idea, rather than waiting until symptoms arise.

------

[6] Lemon essential oil and placebo were given to the intervention and control groups, respectively, to inhale it as soon as they felt nausea. The nausea, vomiting, and retch intensity were investigated 24 hours before and during the four days of treatment. Iran Red Crescent Med J. 2014 Mar;16(3):e14360. doi: 10.5812/ircmj.14360. Epub 2014 Mar 5.

Labor

Some oils can be very helpful for labor:

Symptom	Oils (not exhaustive)
Pain	Frankincense, Lavender & Clary Sage (combined) diluted in carrier oil
Nausea	Peppermint and/or Lemon (inhaled)
Contraction strength	Clary Sage (diluted over lower back)
Placenta delivery	Warm compresses of Clary Sage over abdomen
Stretch marks after delivery	Lavender, Geranium, and Myrrh diluted in Pumpkin seed (carrier oil) applied 2-3 times daily

Which Oils Do I Use for What Purpose?

Below is a list of oils that have been tested and/or have shown in my experience to assist with various concerns. I note that essential oils are *never* meant to replace medical professional advice. Essential oils are also *never* meant to cure a medical condition. Always tell your doctor before using a new alternative health treatment, including essential oils. And of course, always remember to dilute before using topically.

TIP - Remember that essential oils are most effective when used at the <u>first</u> sign of an issue. I can't stress this enough. You can significantly shorten a cold or flu by catching it in the earliest stages.

TIP - For general systemic uses, you should apply diluted oils to feet, spine, or over larger lymph nodes like those in neck and behind the knees (some oils may be more irritating, so the feet may be a better choice for those but generally the feet aren't the best place to use essential oils due to the thickness of the skin.)

When to Inhale or use Topically

When using oils for any of these or other issues, remember that *diffusing* or inhaling the oils is the safest and fastest way to assist with issues like:

- Emotions (anxiety, stress, panic)

- Memory

- Focus

- Killing airborne germs

- Congestion/Cough

However, *topical* uses are best for issues like:

- Acne

- Joint pain

- Muscle pain

- Stomach issues

- Constipation

- Cramps

- Insect bites

- Warts

- Skin issues (rashes, dry skin)

Always remember that dilution is necessary for any topical use. As we have discussed, dilution ratios depend on things like the oil used; the age, ethnicity, and health issues of the individual; and the condition from which you seek relief. The elderly have a more permeable skin reaction as do the very young. Those ethnicities with more pigment many times can tolerate much greater concentration of essential oils.

WHEN TO INHALE, APPLY, OR INGEST YOUR OILS.
A QUICK GUIDE

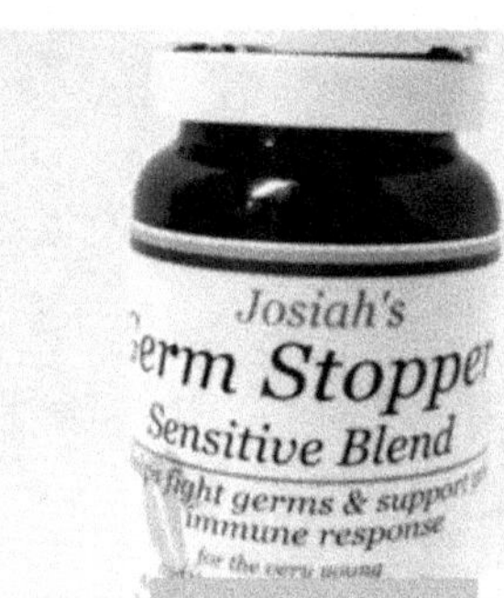

1

WHEN DO YOU DIFFUSE OR INHALE OILS

CONCENTRATION, MEMORY, EMOTIONAL (DEPRESSION/ANXIETY), SLEEP-RELATED, CONGESTION, INTERNAL PAIN, NAUSEA, REFLUX, TO KILL AIRBORNE GERMS

*INHALE WITH A DIFFUSER, PERSONAL INHALER, SNIFFING FROM BOTTLE OR EVEN WEARING OILS

2

WHEN TO APPLY TO THE SKIN

ACNE, JOINT OR MUSCLE PAIN, RASH/ ITCHY SKIN, WARTS, HEADACHE, STOMACH CRAMPS, PMS SYMPTOMS, CONSTIPATION, TO KILL GERMS ON THE SKIN, TO REDUCE WRINKLES OR SCARRING, TO SUPPORT LYMPHATIC SYSTEM

*PROPERLY DILUTE BEFORE YOU APPLY

3

WHEN SHOULD YOU TAKE OIL INTERNALLY?

SYSTEMIC HEALTH ISSUES, WHEN AN OIL HAS **GRAS** STATUS, WHEN YOU ARE WORKING WITH A PROFESSIONAL, TAKING PROPER PRECAUTIONS, AND FOR LIMITED PERIODS OF TIME

The use list below provides the oils that are known to assist with the issues listed, but you obviously do not need to use all of them for each issue.

Try starting with a single oil, or a pre-made blend created by a trained aromatherapist. It is best to start with one oil, rather than a blend, if you tend to be an allergic or sensitive individual. Once you get more comfortable with using essential oils, try creating your own blend with two or three complimentary oils.

When creating a blend, I like to always have a top note, which is a lighter oil like lemon, in my blends along with a middle and/or base note, which simply are heavier essential oils (like frankincense or patchouli). You can get an idea for which oils fall into which note category by smelling them, applying them topically, and seeing how long the scent lingers. We will discuss this is greater detail in the <u>Blending Made Easy</u> Section of this book.

Acne

Sandalwood, Tea Tree, Lavender, May Chang, Rosalina, Copaiba

Balsam (studied to be effective at reducing acne at only a 1%

dilution ratio), Elemi (for oil prone skin), (Josiah's Oils Complete

Acne Blend) (apply topically daily.)

Adrenal Fatigue

Rosemary, Pine, Peppermint, Spearmint, Grapefruit, Geranium,

Lemongrass (diffusing is best; also apply diluted topically over

adrenal gland 2-3 times weekly.)

Anti-inflammatory Oils

Copaiba, Helichrysum, Turmeric, Frankincense, Geranium,

Peppermint, Rosemary, Sandalwood, Tea Tree, Ylang Ylang, Black

Pepper, Myrrh, Vanilla Bean, Josiah's Pain Relief Blend (topically

applied diluted in Jojoba Oil; always include Copaiba or

Helichrysum in your blends for anti-inflammatory issues.)

Anti-Spasmodic Oils

Citronella, Coriander, Ginger, Helichrysum (topically applied

diluted in Jojoba Oil.)

Anxiety

Clary Sage, Lavender, Cedarwood, Ho Wood, Citrus Fruits (like Tangerine, Lemon and Sweet Orange), Ylang Ylang, Valerian, Frankincense, R. Chamomile, Hyssop, Sweet Marjoram, Palmerosa, PaloSanto, Patchouli, Vanilla Bean, Josiah's Peace & Balance, RELAX, Serenity, Kids' Calm, Sleepy Time, Worry Less (diffused is best; also great for a personal inhaler or to wear topically to inhale.) remember to speak with your doctor for medical treatment.)

Arthritis

Frankincense Serrata, Copaiba, Peppermint, Cedarwood, Nutmeg, Ginger, Lavender, Wintergreen, Clove, Aniseed, Josiah's Pain Relief (topically applied diluted in Jojoba Oil.) remember to speak with your doctor for medical treatment.)

Arousal

Ylang Ylang (diffused is best.)

Asthma

Cypress, Frankincense, Eucalyptus, Myrrh, Sandalwood (diffusing is best. Asthma is a serious condition; always consult your physician.)

Attention

Vetiver, Cedarwood, Sweet Orange, Frankincense, (Josiah's FOCUS

Blend) (use diluted on back of neck over brain stem and diffuse.)

Bee Stings

Roman Chamomile, Lavender, Helicrysum, Copaiba, Tea Tree,

(Josiah's Bite Repair) (diluted applied topically is best.)

Boils

Frankincense & Myrrh, Tea Tree, Lavender, Patchouli (dilute in

Coconut Oil for topical use.)

Bruises

Lavender, Frankincense, Helichrysum, Copaiba (apply topically

diluted in Jojoba or Sweet Almond.)

Minor Bleeding

Helichrysum (Topically, but always seek medical help for serious

injuries.)

Bad Breath

Gargle with warm water and Fennel, Peppermint, and/or Myrrh

Bursitis

Basil, Eucalyptus, Lemon, Grapefruit, Roman Chamomile, Cypress,

Juniper, Lavender, Sweet Marjoram, Black pepper, Pine, Rosemary,

Clove, Helichrysum (best applied topically diluted in carrier oil.)

Candida

Patchouli, Tea tree, Clove (with caution), Eucalyptus, Lavender,

(Josiah's Candida Bath Blend) (in bath.)

Canker Sore

Lemon, Cilantro and Tea Tree (apply diluted topically.)

Cellulite

Cypress, Lavender, and Grapefruit (all 3) diluted in Jojoba Oil and

applied topically.

Congestion

Eucalyptus, Peppermint, Lavender, Lemon, Tea Tree, Fir, Pine,

(Josiah's Congestion Blend and Sniffles Blend for younger

children), Lemon Eucalyptus, Sweet Marjoram, Citronella,

Rosalina, Juniper Berry, Oregano (diffusing is always best for

congestion. A diluted chest rub may also be made by adding drops

of essential oil in coconut oil or raw Shea butter.)

Constipation

Fennel, Sweet Orange, Blood Orange, Peppermint, Ginger (select 2

oils but the blend should have Sweet or Blood Orange, dilute and

rub on abdomen.) Also, try Josiah's Digestion Blend.

Cough

(Josiah's Congestion Blend), (Josiah's Sniffles Blend), Ginger, Tea Tree, Lemon, Eucalyptus, Rosalina, Ravensara (diffusing is best, but a chest rub can be made as well (see Congestion).) (remember to speak with your doctor for medical treatment.)

Cramps

Clary Sage or Geranium (diluted in carrier oil of choice and applied over area affected; oils from the Pain category can be used as well.) Serenity Blend works well as well.

Depressed Mood

Lavender, Bergamot, Tangerine, Frankincense, Sweet Orange, Valerian Root, Ho Wood, Josiah's Happiness Blend, Worry Less Blend (diffused is best.) (remember to speak with your doctor for medical treatment.)

Dry skin

Sandalwood, Myrrh, Patchouli, Helichrysum (diluted in Jojoba Oil.)

Dandruff

Lavender, Tea Tree, Cedarwood (added to shampoo or create a scalp serum by adding drops of essential oil to carrier and massaging into scalp.)

Patchouli and Tea Tree (topically diluted in Coconut Oil.)

Benzoin, Elemi, Geranium, Lavender, Frankincense, Roman

Chamomile, Helichrysum, Copaiba Balsam, (Josiah's Skin Rescue)

(diluted and applied topically.)

Cilantro, Lemongrass, Grapefruit, May Chang, Josiah's Immune

Boost (inhale and apply diluted over lymph nodes and liver area.)

Fennel, Juniper, Ginger, Peppermint, Cilantro, Aniseed, Spearmint

(Josiah's Digestion Blend) (diluted- 2 or 3 oils and rub over

stomach; also inhale before and after meals.) (remember to speak

with your doctor for medical treatment.)

Gargle with Grapefruit and Lime using warm water

Elemi, Helichrysum, Lavender, Lemon, Copaiba, Frankincense,

Myrrh, Benzoin, (Josiah's Skin Rescue) (select 2-3 complimentary oils; apply 2-3 oils diluted in jojoba or raw Shea butter 2-3 times

daily.) remember to speak with your doctor for medical treatment.)

Fatigue

Sweet Orange, Rosemary, Basil, Juniper, Pine, Cinnamon,

Grapefruit, Spearmint, Eucalyptus, Black Pepper (diffused in best;

can also be made into a roller bottle to wear throughout the busy

day.)

Fever

Peppermint, Bergamot, Lavender, Lemon (dilute a single oil or

blend on feet and base of neck; can use cool compress.) (remember

to speak with your doctor for medical treatment.)

Fibromyalgia

Black Pepper, Peppermint, Sweet Marjoram, Frankincense,

Copaiba, Sweet Birch, Turmeric, Helichrysum, Lavender (Blend 2 or

3 oils with jojoba and apply diluted topically to areas of pain and

along spine as needed.) Josiah's Pain Relief Blend. remember to

speak with your doctor for medical treatment.)

Amyris (smells similar to sandalwood for far less cost) and

Benzoin (smells like Vanilla for far less cost; use in your blends to

create a stronger, longer lasting scent)

Fennel and Ginger (combine, dilute and rub on stomach.)

(Josiah's Focus Blend), Vetiver, Rosemary, Basil, Lemon, Lemon

Eucalyptus, Peppermint, Grapefruit, Cypress (diffusing is best;

select 2 or 3 oils always including Vetiver.)

Clove or Myrrh (dilution in coconut oil.)

Rosemary, Peppermint, and Cedarwood (diluted in Jojoba or

Grapeseed carrier oil and applied to scalp 2-3 times weekly.)

May Chang (add to shampoo; use 2-3 times per week)

Fennel, Peppermint, Ginger, Sandalwood (dilute and rub on

esophagus.) (see digestion oils as well)

Headache/Migraines

(Josiah's Migraine Relief, Josiah's Headache Roll-on) (both on area of pain as they are pre-diluted), Peppermint, Lavender, Helichrysum, Copaiba (always dilute and avoid eyes; apply to temples or base of back of neck.) (Remember to seek medical treatment when needed.)

Heart Health

Petitgrain, Ylang Ylang, Sweet Orange, Clary Sage, Helichrysum (Dilute and apply topically over vascular areas daily) (remember to speak with your doctor for medical treatment.)

Hemorrhoids

Basil, Clary, Lavender, Copaiba, Frankincense, Helichrysum (diluted and applied topically; witch hazel helps as well.)

Hormone Balance

Clary Sage, Geranium, Josiah's Peace & Balance Blend, Josiah's Serenity Blend (best diffused and applied topically after dilution.)

Hot Flashes

Clary Sage and Peppermint (dilute both and apply down back of neck and spine as needed.)

Hyperactivity

Cedarwood, Vetiver, Lavender, Ho Wood, Sweet Orange, Petitgrain, Josiah's FOCUS Blend, Kids' Calm, Worry Less (diffuse and use diluted applied topically on wrists and neck area.)

IBS

Juniper, Peppermint, Spearmint, Sweet Orange, Fennel, Sweet Marjoram, Ginger, Neroli, (Josiah's Sore Tummy Blend) (dilute up to 3 oils and apply on lower stomach.) (remember to speak with your doctor for medical treatment.)

Immune

Frankincense, Palmarosa, Sandalwood, Josiah's Immune Boost, Josiah's Germ Stopper. (diffuse and apply diluted over lymph nodes) (Oils high in phenols like clove tend to stimulate the immune system.)

Insect Bites

Lavender, Tea Tree, Copaiba, Frankincense, (Josiah's Bite Repair) (dilute to 50% ratio and apply on bite area.)

Insomnia

Bergamot, Lavender, (Josiah's Sleepy Time Blend), Frankincense, Vetiver, Clary Sage, Lemon, Roman Chamomile, Sweet Marjoram,

Juniper, Rose, Palo Santo, Sandalwood, Ylang Ylang, Valerian ,

Josiah's Worry Less. (select 2 or 3 non-blend oils; diffusing is best.)

Joint Pain
(see Anti-inflammatory & Pain)

Lactation
To increase supply use Geranium, Fennel, Basil (Use Peppermint to

decrease milk supply) (best applied topically. Always avoid the

oils coming in contact with the baby.)

Laryngitis
Gargle with Frankincense in warm water. (one or two drops in 1/4

cup of water is sufficient.) (remember to speak with your doctor

for medical treatment.)

Head Lice
Tea Tree and Rosemary (add drops to shampoo or create a serum

by adding essential oil to carrier oil and apply a shower cap and let

sit for 20 minutes before washing off.)

Mental Clarity
Amyris, Rosemary, Lemon, Lime, Spearmint (inhaled)

Clove, Cinnamon, Lemon, Orange, Rosemary, Eucalyptus, Palma Rosa, Tea Tree, (Josiah's Germ Fighting Blend or Germ Stopper for sensitive individuals), Oregano, Thyme, (diffused is best for airborne pathogens; do not diffuse all of these oils at once; use caution with irritating oils.); for scrubbing take 1 cup baking soda add 25 drops essential oils, mix well and scrub - use caution with surfaces!

Ginger, Lemongrass, and Rosemary all blended in Jojoba Oil and massaged. Amyris is also excellent for this diluted at 5% and applied topically.

(Josiah's Cool n' Hot), Wintergreen, Sweet Birch, Peppermint, Sweet Marjoram, Eucalyptus (dilute and apply topically.)

Peppermint, Ginger, Spearmint, Lemon, Fennel, Vanilla, (Josiah's Sore Tummy Blend) (Diffusing is best, also dilute and apply over abdomen.)

Nose Bleed

Inhale Helichrysum and apply topically over bridge of nose. (Seek medical treatment when needed.)

Pain

Peppermint, Black Pepper, Wintergreen, Sweet Birch, Turmeric, Frankincense (Josiah's Pain Relief Roll-On Blend) (apply topically diluted to area 2-3 times daily.)

Panic

Vetiver, Clary Sage, Valerian, Sweet Marjoram, Lavender, Bergamot, Frankincense, (Josiah's Peace & Balance or Worry Less) (Diffusing is best; great to carry in a personal inhaler to use as needed.) (remember to speak with your doctor for medical treatment.)

PMS

Geranium, Clary Sage, Frankincense, (Josiah's Peace & Balance) (diffuse and apply topically.)

Poor Circulation

Basil, Eucalyptus, Grapefruit, Lemon, Sweet Orange, Cinnamon, Black Pepper, Ginger, Turmeric, Rosemary, Clove, Nutmeg (dilute 2 or 3 essential oils and massage on extremities.)

Muscle Spasms

Sweet Marjoram, Ginger, Peppermint, Lavender, Eucalyptus

(diluted in Jojoba Oil and massaged.)

Muscle strain

Lavender, Ginger, Peppermint, Wintergreen, Sweet Marjoram,

(Josiah's Cool n' Hot Blend) (diluted and applied topically -

especially with massage.)

Nail Fungus

Tea Tree Oil, Oregano, Lemon (Josiah's Nail Fugal Serum) (diluted

well and applied on nail 2-3 times daily.)

Tinnitus

Peppermint and Copaiba (diluted together and applied behind the

ears.)

SAD

Sweet Orange, Tangerine, Lemon, Lime, Bergamot, Frankincense,

(Josiah's Oils Happiness Blend) (diffusing is best.) *Always consult

a physician for mental health issues.

Skin (wrinkles)

Coffee Bean (firming), Carrot Seed, Myrrh, Elemi, Rose (Josiah's Anti-Aging Serum) (applied topically diluted blend in Pumpkin Seed Carrier oil due to its high anti-oxidant content.)

Sleep Apnea

Vanilla bean (inhaled) (remember to speak with your doctor for medical treatment.)

Sore throat

Gargle with diluted Sandalwood and Bergamot in warm water.

Urinary Issues

Sitz bath with Tea Tree and Lavender (may add Bergamot)

Varicose Veins

Diluted Cypress applied topically 2-3 times daily.

Viruses

Sandalwood, Hyssop, Thyme, Eucalyptus, Tea Tree (Diffuse and apply diluted over major lymph nodes especially at first sign of illness.) (remember to speak with your doctor for medical treatment.)

Vomiting

Fennel, Peppermint, Ginger (diffused and applied topically over stomach.)

Tea Tree, Lemon, Oregano (topical with 1:1 dilution using care to avoid getting oils on surrounding skin.)

Peppermint , Grapefruit, Lemongrass, Josiah's Curb Blend (diffused is best. This blend is perfect for your personal inhaler.)

Some More Hopeful Studies of Essential Oils

Like mentioned earlier, the health care industry is starting to provide more research providing further proof of the benefits of essential oils. For example, a 2016 study showed that Lavender aromatherapy had beneficial effects on pain, anxiety, and satisfaction level of patients undergoing surgery.[7]

In a 2013 article, researchers at Xiamen University, China, concluded:

"Most studies, as well as clinically applied experience, have indicated that various essential oils, such as lavender, lemon and

---

[7] Copyright © 2016 Elsevier Ltd. All rights reserved.
http://www.ncbi.nlm.nih.gov/pubmed/27157961

bergamot can help to relieve stress, anxiety, depression and other mood disorders. Most notably, inhalation of essential oils can communicate signals to the olfactory system and stimulate the brain to exert neurotransmitters (e.g. serotonin and dopamine) thereby further regulating mood."[8]

With regard to mood, many us us have heard about the devastating health effects of prolonged stress. Cortisol - known as the stress hormone - can remain elevated over time causing:

• Anxiety

• Depression

• Digestive problems

• Heart disease

• Sleep problems

• Weight gain

• Memory and concentration impairment

• Diabetes

---

[8] http://www.ncbi.nlm.nih.gov/pubmed/23531112.

• Hair loss

A very impressive study from 2014 examined the antidepressant-like effects of Clary Sage oil on human beings by comparing the neurotransmitter level change in blood plasma. Here voluntary participants were 22 menopausal women in their 50's. After inhalation of Clary Sage oil, cortisol levels were "significantly decreased" in the participants. The conclusion was that "Clary Sage oil has antidepressant-like effect."[9]

Some oils can offer stimulating properties. Black pepper is one of the only essential oils that has been shown to significantly increase epinephrine levels on inhalation (Haze et al 2002) and so might be useful where lethargy is a problem, but perhaps not if anxiety is high. Also in healthy adults, inhaled grapefruit oil can be stimulating and invigorating, increasing the activity of the sympathetic nervous system by 50%, and causing a slight increase in skin temperature (Haze et al 2002). Grapefruit oil inhalation

[9] http://www.ncbi.nlm.nih.gov/pubmed/24802524

slightly increased epinephrine and norepinephrine levels. The effect was not statistically significant, but it may reveal a tendency. (Haze et al 2002).

Back to Clary, in my practice, I have seen amazing results from combining clary sage with other oils known to induce a relaxed state of mind, like frankincense. Many of my clients carry a personal inhaler in their purse or briefcase to sniff throughout the day, especially when times get stressful. I note that clary sage can lower blood pressure in some people, so take care if you generally experience low blood pressure.

I once made myself a powerful relaxing blend to inhale during a flight as flying can make me extremely anxious. I combined valerian root with frankincense and a light oil of Sweet Orange. It worked beautifully! I commonly make a relaxing perfume-alternative for clients with a combination of Ylang Ylang and Vanilla in a carrier oil such as jojoba. Simple & effective!

Back to the scientific studies, another study showed the antidepressant-like effect of inhaled clary sage while testing the dopamine levels in rats undergoing forced swim tasks.[10] While the human study was most impressive, this study supports the concept that clary sage may help when we are asked to perform under pressure.

A very encouraging study involved postpartum women and the symptoms of stress, anxiety, and depression during the months following delivery. The study concluded that inhalation of lavender essential oil can lead to <u>prevention of stress, anxiety, and postpartum depression</u>, it can be used as a complementary method to prevent these disorders! This study noted that the longevity of aromatherapy increased the therapeutic benefits, which is a fact I have experienced in my practice as well. [11]

---

[10] Copyright (c) 2010 Elsevier Ireland Ltd. All rights reserved.

[11] www.ncbi.nlm.nih.gov/pmc/articles/PMC4815377/

A personal favorite oil of mine was the subject of some recent studies as well. Copaiba balsam essential oil is commonly featured in anti-inflammatory recipes. In one study, copaiba was noted for its anti-inflammatory and neuroprotective agents following an acute damage to a patient's central nervous system.[12]

With regard to acne, copaiba oil has proven extremely effective with significant reduction in acne at just a 1% dilution ratio (1 drop of copaiba in 1 teaspoon of carrier; for acne a lighter oil like grapeseed is a good carrier choice.)[13]

Another hopeful study featured peppermint essential oil. Traditionally used for stomach issues and for congestion, this oil proved effective against hair loss. Researchers stated:

"In conclusion, our experimental data suggest that 3% [peppermint essential oil] facilitates hair growth by promoting the conservation of vascularization of hair dermal papilla, which may contribute to the induction of early anagen stage. In addition, PEO

---

[12] http://www.ncbi.nlm.nih.gov/pmc/articles/PMC3291111/

[13] http://www.ncbi.nlm.nih.gov/pubmed/22502624

effectively stimulated hair growth in an animal model via several mechanisms and thus could be used as a therapeutic or preventive alternative medicine for hair loss in humans"[14] Thus, making a scalp serum with only a 3% concentration of peppermint oil in a carrier oil may help those who suffer hair loss.

Of course studies support the most common uses of peppermint oil as well. For example, peppermint is an excellent choice to reduce nausea - even post-operative nausea.[15] With regard to irritable bowel syndrome, another human study found peppermint essential oil "significantly superior to placebo for global improvement of IBS symptoms." [16] For these types of conditions, remember that both inhalation and (properly diluted) topical applications are best. I often diffuse peppermint in my car diffuser for long car trips to avoid motion sickness and tiredness.

[14] http://www.ncbi.nlm.nih.gov/pmc/articles/PMC4289931/

[15] http://www.ncbi.nlm.nih.gov/pubmed/22392970
Another post-operative use study: http://www.ncbi.nlm.nih.gov/pubmed/22034523

[16] http://www.ncbi.nlm.nih.gov/pubmed/24100754

You can make it even more effective by adding a few drops of lemon to the diffuser as well. Lemon and Peppermint make a delicious-smelling trip!

Another study showed hope for Sleep Apnea. A study tested 36 pre-mature infants by placing a cotton ball with of 2% saturated solution of vanillin - found in Vanilla oil. The study showed that diffusing Vanilla Oil in this manner could "significantly decrease apnea through the newborns' olfactory stimulation. Thus, it can be concluded that vanillin saturated solution might decrease the incidence of apnea in premature newborns and, at the same time, protect them against the dangerous complications of the disease." https://www.ncbi.nlm.nih.gov/pmc/articles/PMC3684469/

Next, there is always much talk about "DeToxing" in essential oils use groups! I often see products that claim oils "Detox" the body, but how do they work and do they really work at all? Detoxification is "the metabolic process by which toxins are changed into less toxic or more readily excrete-able substances."

The body excretes via Kidneys (urine), Lungs (exhaled), and Skin as well as the lower intestines.

Your body was designed by God to naturally remove toxins. Unfortunately, our toxic overload is only increasing. Polluted air, dangerous bath and body products, the water supply, food additives and pesticides are only a few we are commonly exposed to. In the specialty of essential oils, I have seen powerful body function assistance with using the correct oil in the correct way. Looking closely, we see that some oils can assist the body's *natural elimination process* of undesirable substances along by stimulation things like the lymphatic system, lungs, and liver.

Your body naturally excretes things like mucus to release toxic matter for example. Therefore an expectorant oil like eucalyptus assists the body's detoxification process. Other examples of our body's natural defenses include the lymphatic system which naturally acts to clean the tissue of toxins and the liver function which detoxifies the body.

There are quite a few oils exceptionally high in antioxidants which will naturally assist the body's natural excretion and detoxification function. Antioxidants help prevent or stop cell damage caused by oxidants. One such oil is May Chang, which contains over 65% citral! Another example is Lemongrass, which contains over 75% citral - an extraordinary oil constituent to assist the body's natural detoxification process.

<u>TIP</u>- You may simply add Add 4-6 drops of two citral-rich oils in your diffuser daily!

<u>TIP</u> - Adding a few drops of Peppermint helps enhance the antioxidant dosage and creates an excellent odor killing scent as well! You may also dilute an oil like May Chang in Golden Jojoba Oil and apply to your lymph nodes to assist natural detoxification.

An excellent blend to cleanse the body and support the immune system is the Immune Boost Blend, which also contains powerful anti-inflammatories to help reduce lymphatic congestion. (Always speak with your doctor first if you are under treatment.) Oils in the Immune Boost assist the body in the following ways:

Studies have demonstrated that <u>Frankincense</u> has immune-enhancing abilities that may help the body's ability to destroy bacteria and viruses. It can even be used to prevent germs from forming on the skin.

<u>Palma Rosa</u> has been studied to be an agent against both gram negative and gram positive bacteria (https://www.ncbi.nlm.nih.gov/pmc/articles/PMC2839398/)

<u>Lemon</u> oil is high vitamin content, making it valuable for the body's immune system. It further stimulates white blood cells, thus increasing your ability to fight off diseases. Lemon oil also improves circulation throughout the body!

Next, <u>Copaiba</u> is a strong antibacterial that can act as a major booster for your immune system. It can act as a shield for your skin, protecting any irritations (not open wounds) from developing an infection. It also protects you by eliminating harmful bacteria and viruses and by reducing inflammation throughout the body.

Finally, <u>Lavender</u> essential oil is a natural antioxidant that works to prevent disease. A 2013 study published in <u>Phytomedicine</u> stated that lavender oil increased the activity of the body's most powerful antioxidants — glutathione, catalase, and SOD.   Recent studies have indicated similar results, concluding that lavender has antioxidant activity and helps to prevent or reverse oxidative stress.

A side note, redness and irritation is NEVER a sign of detoxification from an essential oil. If an oil irritates the skin, stop using it and seek medical help if necessary.

This brings us to an area of great interest for many, antibiotic resistant bacteria, such as MRSA. The following essential oils have been shown effective against MRSA: Tea Tree Oil, Lemongrass, True Lavender (Spike and Spanish Lavenders as well), Geranium, Eucalyptus, Garlic. Oils shown effective against E. Coli include: Palma Rosa, Oregano, Sweet Orange, Bergamot, Lemon, Lemongrass, Eucalyptus, Clary Sage, True Lavender, and Ylang Ylang. Oils shown to be effective against Streptococcus include Peppermint, Eucalyptus, and Lemongrass. These studies provide hope for the future as antibiotic resistance is becoming the "new norm".

Also interesting is the use of essential oils to aid in stopping the spread of mosquito-born illness such as Malaria and West Nile Virus. Spearmint essential oil has been shown to be toxic against larvae of three types of mosquitos. (Govindarajan et al 2012.) We hope to see more studies that show the effectiveness of essential oils used to prevent these diseases and do away with antibiotic resistance as well.

Lastly, I have compiled a list of many essential oils that have proven analgesic (pain relieving) components:

Spearmint, Black Pepper, Lemongrass, Eucalyptus, Clove, Clary Sage, Fennel, Leon Eucalyptus, True Lavender, Lemon, peppermint, Basil, Rosemary, Thyme, Tea Tree, and Sweet Marjoram.

Several OTC drugs also have analgesic components, but also have more serious side effects than many essential oils including being taxing on the liver. For those experiencing pain, always try to couple analgesic oils with anti-inflammatory oils many of which are listed in this book. And always discuss adding essential oils to your plan with your medical doctor. Next, we will take a brief look at some of the more common essential oils you may wish to start your collection with.

Lavender (*Lavandula angustifolia*)

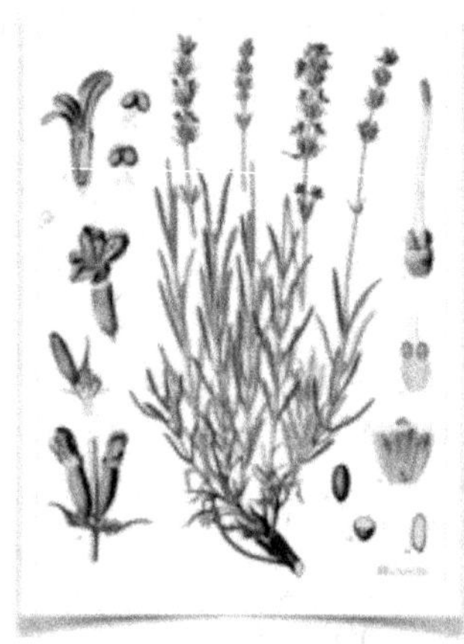

<u>Properties</u>:
Calming
Pain Relieving
Anti-Bacterial
Anti-Histamine
Anti-Bacterial
<u>Common Use Ideas</u>:
Inhale for allergies
Dilute and massage for headache (1-2% for head avoiding eyes)
Dilute and apply to minor cuts
Diffuse for calming/sleep
Make a room mist for relaxation
Dilute and apply to sore muscles

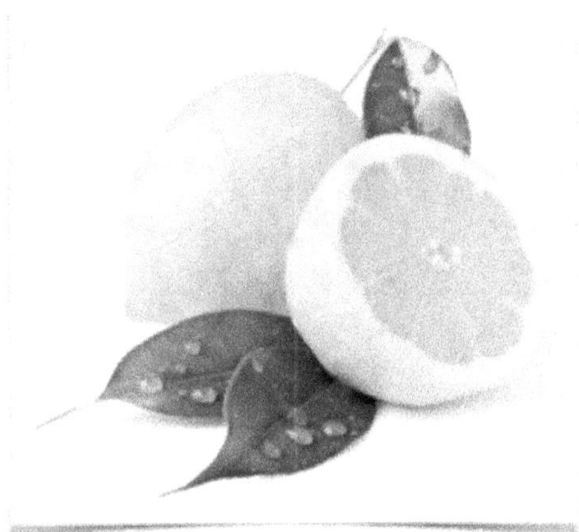

Properties:
Cooling
Cleansing
Disinfecting
Detoxifying
Anti-nausea
Analgesic
Common Use Ideas:
Diffuse for mood or to purify the air
Place in a spray bottle for cleaning (10% dilution ratio-
shake well with each use)
Inhale in personal inhaler for morning sickness
Apply diluted over liver area
(use caution in the sun)

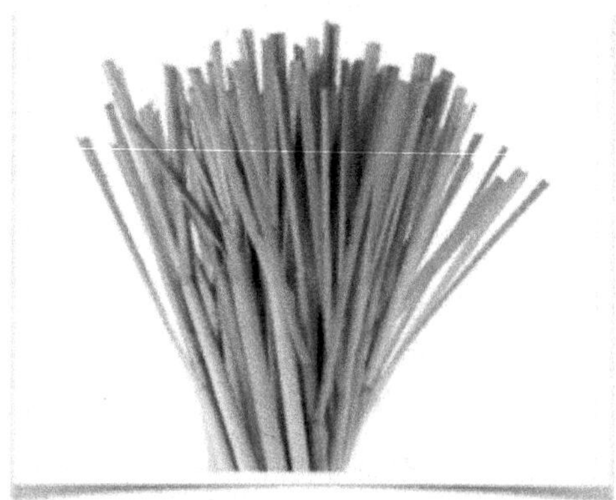

<u>Properties</u>:
Stimulating
Reviving
Insect Repelling
Antiseptic
Analgesic
Aids with congestion
<u>Common Use Ideas</u>:
Diluted to make an insect spray
Diffuse for fatigue or congestion
Dilute and apply topically for pain relief (max. dilution for Lemongrass is .70%)

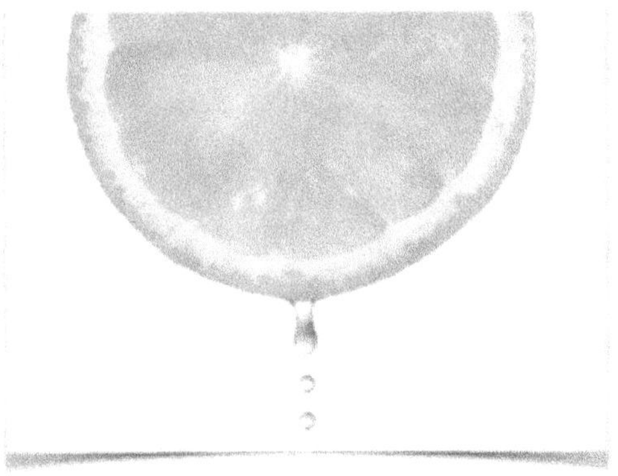

Properties:
Uplifting
Anti-Bacterial
Cheerful
Helps with constipation
Common Use Ideas:
Diffuse for mood
Dilute and massage to lower stomach
Dilute and massage for immune support

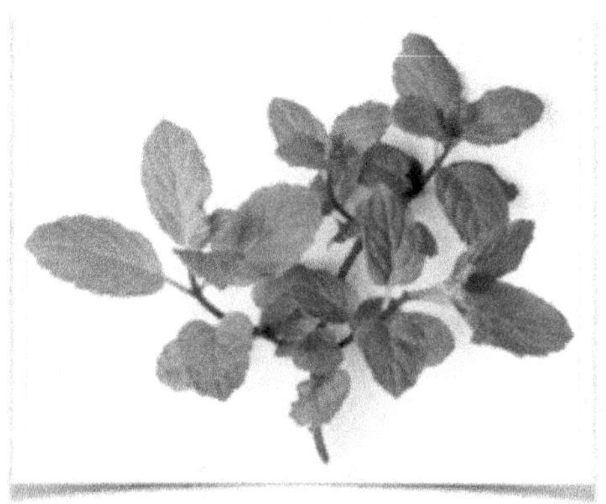

<u>Properties</u>:
Anti-Nausea
Pain Reliever
Anti-Bacterial
Stimulating
Relieves Congestion
<u>Common Use Ideas</u>:
Diffuse
Dilute and massage on stomach (5% dilution ratio)
Dilute and massage for headache (1-2% for head avoiding eyes)
*use with caution on young children

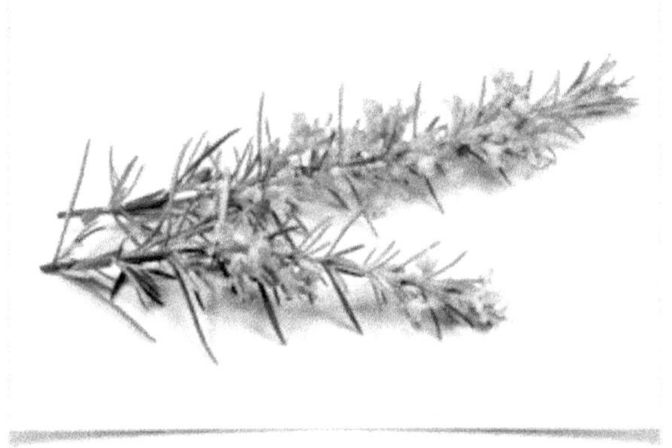

Properties:

Assists with memory

Improves circulation

Anti-Microbial

Aids with Congestion

Analgesic

Common Use Ideas:

Diffuse for memory or congestion

Massage after dilution (max. 5% dilution ratio)

*Use with caution if you have high blood pressure, seizure disorder, when pregnant, and on the very young.

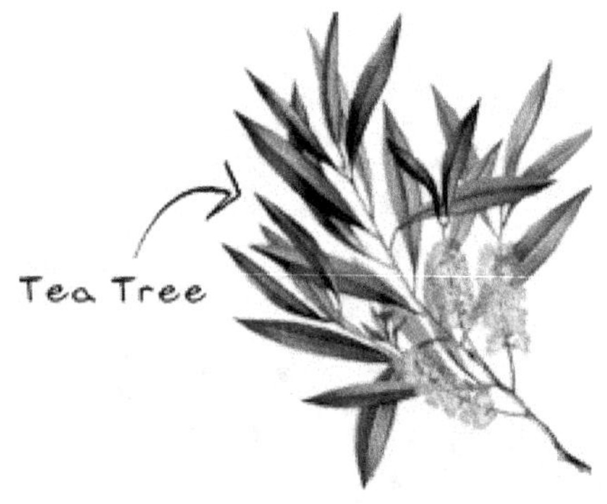

<u>Properties</u>:
Anti-Viral
Anti-Bacterial
Anti-Fungal
Insect Repellent (excellent for lice)
<u>Common use Ideas</u>:
Diffused for viruses and mold
Topically diluted at max. 5% for yeast issues
Topically diluted for warts and nail fungus
*do not ingest Tea Tree Oil

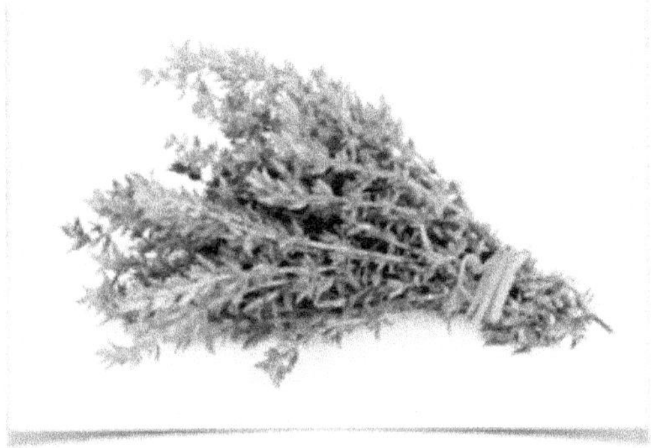

<u>Properties</u>:
Anti-Microbial
Assisting Lungs (commonly used for cold & flu symptoms)
Supporting Immune System
Analgesic

<u>Common Use Ideas</u>:
Diffuse in Water Mist Diffuser at 2% dilution as Thyme is a "hot" oil
Dilute and apply topically to feet (1% dilution maximum)
*use with caution if you have high blood pressure

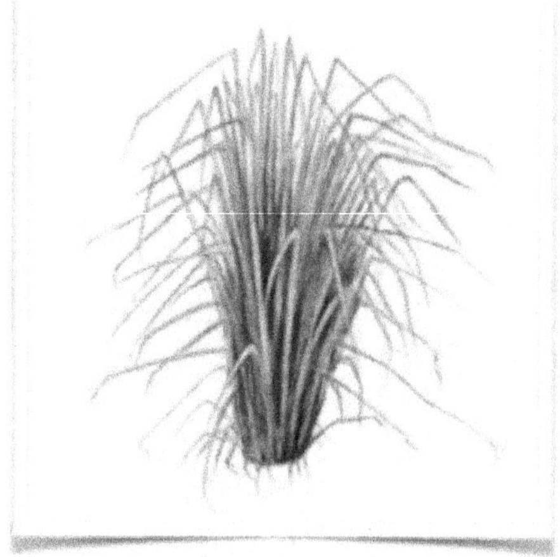

<u>Properties</u>:
Calming
Focusing
Clarifying
Hormone Balance
Assists with oil absorption

<u>Common Use Ideas</u>:
Diffuse or place in personal inhaler for attention, focus,
and concentration issues
Dilute to 5% and massage topically

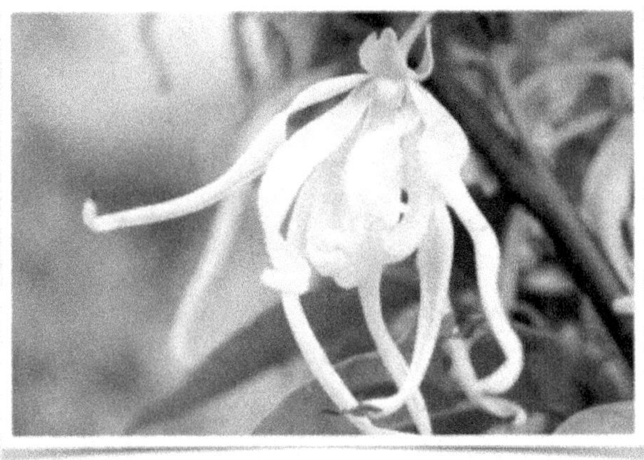

<u>Properties</u>:
Relaxing to nervous system
Excellent for reducing fear, anxiety, and tension.
excellent for arousal

<u>Common Uses</u>:
Diffuse and dilute for topical use (Max. 2% dilution ratio
as can be irritating to the skin)
Use with caution with children

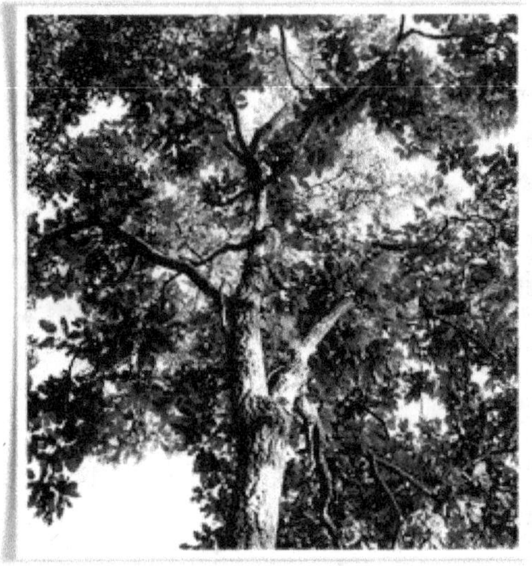

Properties:

Antiseptic
Expectorant for the respiratory tract
Excellent anti-inflammatory
Gentle

Uses:

Diffuse
Dilute and apply to skin (20% dilution for pain; 5% dilution ratio for skin issues)

Now that we have covered safety issues and common uses, let's look into how you <u>can make your own personal blend</u>! The first thing you need to know is how your chosen oil is classified into what is called a note. There are three: Top, Middle, and Base; these classifications are based upon the oils' evaporation rates. The following are examples of each classification:

Top Notes

Basil
Bay Laurel
Bergamot
Citronella
Eucalyptus
Grapefruit
Lavender
Lemon
Lemongrass
Lime
Orange
Peppermint

Petitgrain
Spearmint
Tangerine

Middle Notes

Carrot Seed
Chamomile, German
Chamomile, Roman
Cinnamon
Clary Sage
Clove Bud
Cypress
Fennel
Fir Needle
Geranium
Ho Wood
Hyssop
Jasmine
Juniper Berry
Marjoram
Neroli
Nutmeg
Palmarosa
Parsley
Pepper, Black
Pine, Scotch
Rose
Rose Geranium
Rosemary
Rosewood
Spruce
Tea Tree
Thyme

Yarrow
Ylang Ylang

Benzoin
Cedarwood

Frankincense
Ginger
Helichrysum (Immortelle)
Myrrh

Patchouli
Sandalwood
Vanilla
Vetiver
Valerian

To make your own blend using an oil from each category,

simply start by using this formula for creating your blend:

30% Top Note
50% Middle Note
20% Base Note
(See Quick Guide at end of book)

If you are only using two oils for your blend, choose a Top Note and add either a Middle or Base Note, recalculating as needed as follows:

50% Top Note & 50% Middle Note

80% Top Note and 20% Base Note

If you are creating a pre-diluted blend in a carrier oil, first calculate your dilution ratio, which will generally be 5% as discussed. Thus, per teaspoon of carrier oil, you will have 5 drops of your blend. For a 10 ml bottle (2 teaspoons), you will need 10 drops of your blend! If you are using a per drop recipe instead of a pre-mixed blend, you may then use this recipe:

3 drops of your Top Note
5 drops of your Middle Note
2 drops of your Base Note
2 teaspoons of your carrier oil of choice

OR

8 drops of your Top Note
2 drops of your Base Note

2 teaspoons carrier oil of choice

OR

5 drops of your Top Note
5 drops of your Middle Note
2 teaspoons carrier oil of choice

An example would be:

3 drops Lemon
5 drops Lavender
2 drops Patchouli
2 teaspoons Golden Jojoba Oil

Once you come up with you own blending ideas be sure to write them down and save your favorites; you can give them fun names too - Like Grandma's Boo Boo Spray, Jill's Stuffy Nose Blend. But a more detailed look at blending asks: what is the intended outcome of your blend? You may wish to select oils to address a range of issues. Let me explain this better.

Consider you are having difficulty sleeping as many of us do. You also have been battling with lack of hormonal balance in your life. Thus, you could make a single blend to address both issues by looking at the oils use list for oils that fall into each category you would like help with. Sleep for example, can be aided with Bergamot and hormonal issues with Clary Sage and/or Geranium. These oils can also be used for relaxation, so one blend can help with both issues! Try to select oils from different note categories when possible.

<u>TIP</u> - always try to add a Citrus Oil to your blends to aid in penetration of oils into your system due to their limonene content.

<u>TIP</u> - be sure to write down you blends so you can easy reference them at a later date:

<u>TIP</u> - When blending be sure to let a new blend sit for a few hours or even a day or two to make sure you love it. The scent of the oils changes over time!

<u>TIP</u> - Store your blend in a dark, air-tight glass container to best preserve your blend.

Finally, essential oils can be added to salves for uses on the body, such as vapor rubs or sore muscle rubs. To make a salve use the following recipe:

2 parts Un-bleached, pure beeswax
2 parts Golden Jojoba Oil
2 parts Almond Oil (or Pumpkin Seed Oil)

2 Parts Grapeseed Oil

Heat over double broiler slowly, stirring frequently. Pour into clean glass containers and add essential oils when the salve has cooled, stirring again well. For most blends, remain at a <u>maximum</u> 5 % dilution ratio. If you are filling a 2 ounce glass jar (60 ml or 12 teaspoons), simply add no more than 60 drops of your blend. Again, for younger kids or more sensitizing oils, use a much greater dilution. For example, a 1% dilution means you would add about 12 drops or your essential oil or blend.

For an easy-to-follow Lip Balm Recipe which can be adjusted to make "your own", see the Lip Recipe Guide in the back of this book.

Conclusion (Last thoughts)

Common complaints like hair loss, nausea, depression, stress, and acne are issues many of us face at one time or another. I am so thankful that help can be found naturally in essential oils.

There are several other scientific studies showing the effectiveness of essential oils. I encourage you to research the database at the National Institute of Health to find many more studies exploring the benefits of essential oils on various health concerns. Simply go to PUBMED and click the search bar. Latin or botanical names are usually helpful to select just the right oil needed. These names should be on your individual essential oil bottles. (We always provide them at Josiah's Oils.)

Always consult with your doctor when you decide to add essential oils to help with any health concern for which you are being treated. Finally, consult your trained aromatherapist to learn proper dilution for your oil and any contradictions [interactions] with any medications or allergies. Please feel free to contact us at Josiah's Oils with any questions. Our contact information can be found on our

website: www.josiahsoils.com.

Quick Guide

INHALED OILS
TO NOSE
TO LUNGS
OLFACTORY SYSTEM
BLOOD STREAM
LIMBIC SYSTEM NERVOUS SYSTEM/EMOTIONS/ MEMORY
HORMONE REACTION ABSORPTION INTO TISSUES AND ORAGNS
Josiah's Oils

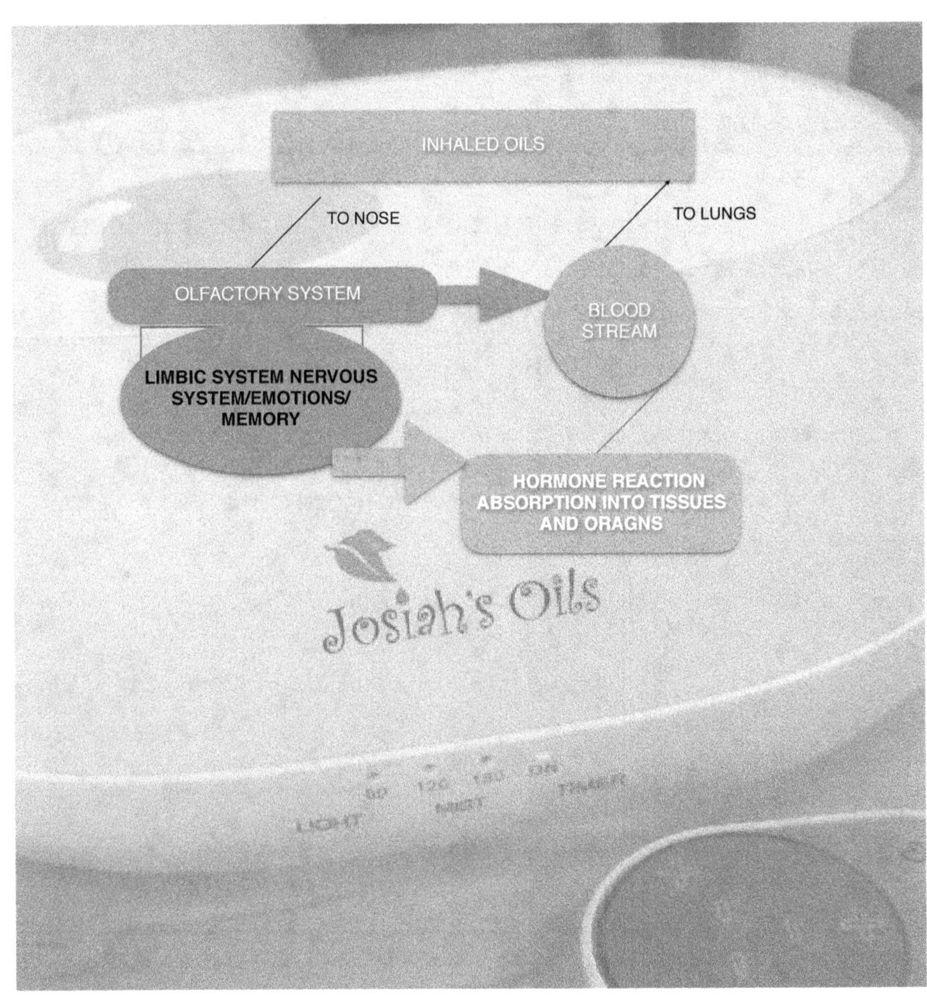

<u>INHALATION AND DIFFUSING GUICK GUIDE</u>

Simply take deep inhalations out of bottle

Tent (always avoid the eyes) or Shower Steam

Palm Inhalations

Use Aroma Sticks

**Use a Diffuser
(water mist or atomizing)**

Josiah's Oils

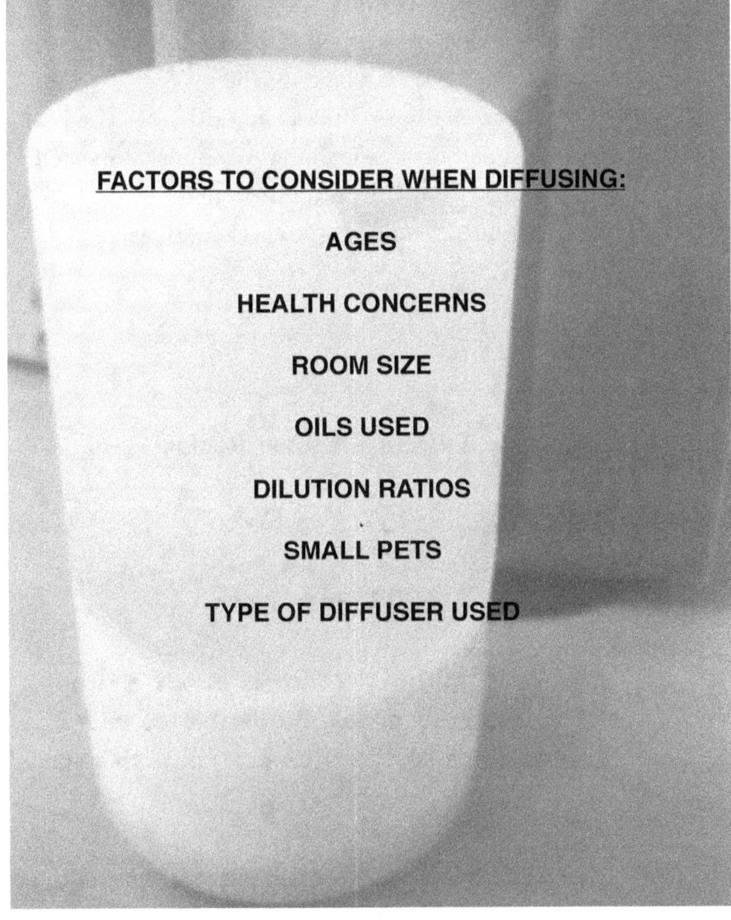

FACTORS TO CONSIDER WHEN DIFFUSING:

AGES

HEALTH CONCERNS

ROOM SIZE

OILS USED

DILUTION RATIOS

SMALL PETS

TYPE OF DIFFUSER USED

Lip Balm -
YUMMY LIPS RECIPE:

1 Tablespoon Raw Shea
enough beeswax to hold (about 1 teaspoon)
2 Teaspoons raw honey
5 drops vanilla bean EO
heat Shea and Bees' Wax in double Boiler; mix well
add oils after heated
pour into empty lip balm containers

Typical Blending Recipe

30% Top Note
50% Middle Note
20% Base Note

For a 10 ml bottle that is about 3 drops
Top Note; 5 drops Middle Note; and 2
drops Base Note; the rest fill with your
carrier oil

*drops may be added based on oils used,
but this is a starting recipe!

General Dilutions Guidelines:
Face - 1% to 2% or less
Body - Maximum 5% (with exceptions)
Pain - Body - Max. 20% (with exceptions)
Small Children - Start at .25% (under 6
Max. 2%)
Elderly - 1% or less to start

1

COMMON GRAS OILS (From FDA)*

Anise
Basil
Bergamot
R. Chamomile
Carrot
Cassia
Cinnamon (Leaf & Bark)
Citronella
Clary Sage
Coffee
Coriander
Fennel
Geranium
Rose Geranium
Ginger
Grapefruit
Hyssop
Helichrysum
Juniper
Laurel Leaf
Lavender
Lemon
Lemongrass

Lime
Sweet Marjoram
Nutmeg
Orange
Oregano
Palmarosa
Black pepper
Peppermint
Petitgrain
Rose
Rosemary
Sage
Spearmint
Tangerine
Thyme
Turmeric
Vanilla
Yang Ylang

*for food flavoring

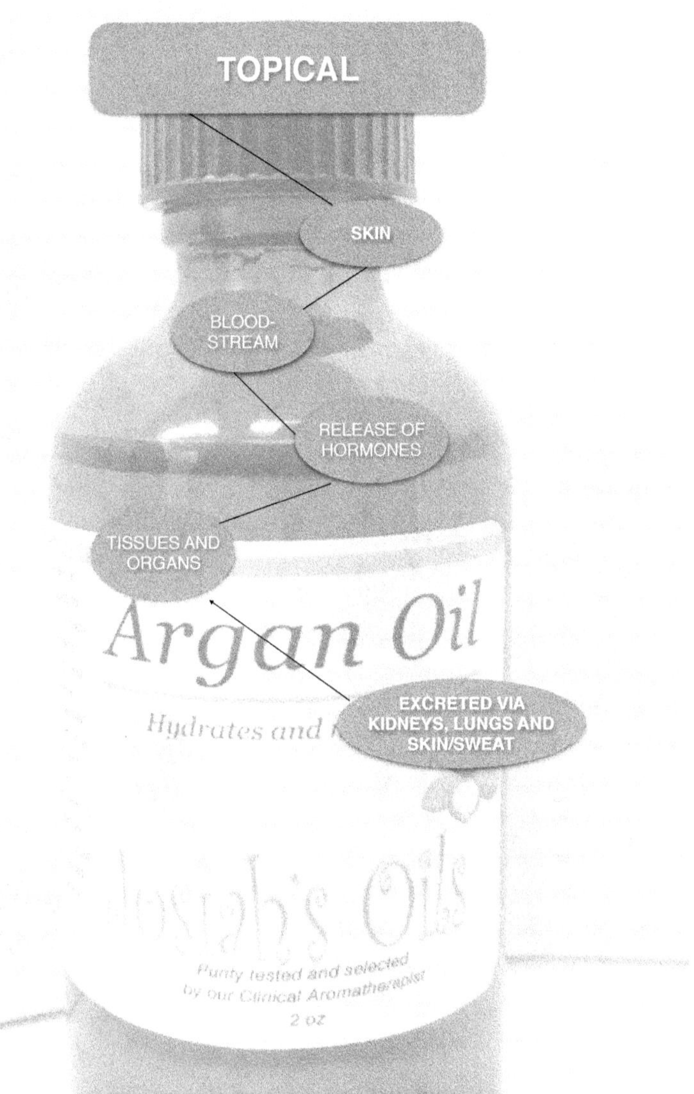

TOPICAL
SKIN
BLOOD-STREAM
RELEASE OF HORMONES
TISSUES AND ORGANS
EXCRETED VIA KIDNEYS, LUNGS AND SKIN/SWEAT
Argan Oil
Hydrates and
Joseph's Oils
Purity tested and selected
by our Clinical Aromatherapist
2 oz

A FEW EASY RECIPE IDEAS

Lavender Lemon Granola Bars

Ingredients
- 2 1/2 cups old rolled oats
- 1/2 cup nuts, roughly chopped
- 1/4 cup honey
- 1/4 cup unsalted butter
- 1/3 cup brown sugar
- 1/4 teaspoon kosher salt
- 3/4 cups total extra mix-ins like dried fruit
- Drops of Lavender and Lemon Oils

1 Preheat the oven to 350 degrees. Line a 9-inch square baking dish with parchment and lightly spray with cooking spray.
2 Place the oats and nuts on a rimmed baking sheet and bake for 8-10 minutes until lightly toasted. Place the nuts and oats in a large bowl.
3 While the oats are toasting, add the honey, butter, and brown sugar to a small saucepan. Cook over medium heat until the butter melts and the sugar dissolves, stirring occasionally. When butter mixture is ready, remove it from the heat and stir in the salt. At this point add your Flavoring Oil; mix 1 drop Lavender and 3 drops Lemon. Pour this mixture over the oat and nut mixture and stir to combine. Add any extra ingredients like dried fruit and stir to combine.
4 Place all of the oat mixture in the prepared pan. Use a rubber spatula or the bottom of a greased measuring cup to press the mixture into the pan. Chill the bars for at least 2 hours. Lift the bars from the pan using the edges of parchment and place them on a cutting board. Cut into desired shape/sizes and serve.

<u>*Crunchy Lime Yogurt*</u>

1 cup ORGANIC Greek yogurt
1/2 cup organic granola
1 drop Lime essential oil in 1 tablespoon honey
Mix Lime oil in honey <u>well</u> then mix in remaining ingredients

<u>*Fall Spice Cookies*</u>

Mix 1 drop Clove, 1 drop Cinnamon, and 1 drop Ginger in your favorite fall cookie recipe calling for molasses (add the oils to molasses and mix well <u>before</u> adding to cookie mix).